Choose life over BREAST CANCER:

A comprehensive Guide to breast cancer.

By Excel shine

Table of content

Chapter 1

What is breast cancer

Breast cancer is a malignant growth that is created in bosom cells. Commonly, the disease structures in either the lobules or the channels of the bosom.

Lobules are the organs that produce milk, and conduits are the pathways that carry the milk from the organs to the areola. The disease can likewise happen in the greasy tissue or the stringy connective tissue inside your bosom.

The uncontrolled disease cells frequently attack other sound bosom tissue and can go to the lymph hubs under the arms. When the disease enters the lymph hubs, it approaches a pathway to move to different pieces of the body.

Cancer happens when changes called transformations occur in qualities that manage cell development. The transformations let the partition and duplicate in an uncontrolled malignant

Chapter2

Symptoms and signs of breast cancer

In its beginning phases, breast Cancer growth may not bring about any side effects. Generally speaking, growth might be excessively little to be felt, however, an irregularity can in any case be seen on a mammogram.

On the off chance that growth can be felt, the principal sign is typically another irregularity in the bosom that was not there previously. Be that as it may, not all irregularities are malignant growth.

Each kind of breast cancer growth can cause different side effects. A significant number of these side effects are comparative, however, some can be unique. Side effects for the most widely recognized breast cancer growths include:

a bosom protuberance or tissue thickening that feels unique about encompassing tissue and is new
bosom torment
red or stained, pitted skin on the bosom
enlarging taking all things together or part of your bosom
an areola release other than bosom milk
horrendous release from your areola
stripping, scaling, or chipping of skin on your areola or breast
an unexpected, unexplained change in the shape or size of your breast
transformed areola
changes to the presence of the skin on your breast
a protuberance or expanding under your arm

On the off chance that you have any of these side effects, it doesn't be guaranteed to mean you have breast cancer growth. For example, torment in your bosom or a bosom irregularity can be brought about by a harmless blister

Early signs of breast cancer

From the beginning, an individual might see an adjustment of their bosom when they play out a month-to-month bosom test or when minor unusual torment doesn't appear to disappear. Early indications of bosom disease to search for include:

changes looking like the areola
bosom torment that doesn't disappear after your next period

another irregularity that doesn't disappear after your next period
areola release from one bosom that is clear, red, brown, or yellow
unexplained redness, expanding, skin disturbance, irritation, or rash on the bosom
enlarging or a protuberance around the collarbone or under the arm
A knot that is hard with unpredictable edges is bound to be dangerous

Later signs of breast cancer

Later signs of breast cancer include:

- withdrawal, or internal turning of the areola
- broadening of one bosom
- dimpling of the bosom surface
- a current irregularity that gets greater

- an "orange strip" surface to the skin
- unfortunate craving
- inadvertent weight reduction
- broadened lymph hubs in the armpit
- noticeable veins on the bosom
- Having at least one of these side effects doesn't guarantee you have bosom malignant growth. Areola release, for instance, can likewise be brought about by disease. See a specialist for a total assessment on the off chance that you experience any of these signs and side effect
-

r

There are a few kinds of bosom disease, and they're broken into two primary classifications: obtrusive and painless. Painless bosom disease is otherwise called bosom malignant growth in situ.

While the obtrusive disease has spread from the bosom conduits or organs to different pieces of the bosom, painless malignant growth has not spread from the first tissue.

These two classifications are utilized to portray the most well-known kinds of bosom malignant growth, which include:

Ductal carcinoma in situ. Ductal carcinoma in situ (DCIS) is a painless condition. With DCIS, the malignant growth cells are bound to the pipes in your bosom and haven't attacked the encompassing bosom tissue.

Lobular carcinoma in situ. Lobular carcinoma in situ (LCIS) is a malignant growth that fills in the milk-delivering organs of your bosom. Like DCIS, the malignant growth cells haven't attacked the encompassing tissue.

Obtrusive ductal carcinoma. Obtrusive ductal carcinoma (IDC) is the most well-known sort of bosom malignant growth. This kind of bosom malignant growth starts in your bosom's milk conduits and afterward attacks close to tissue in the bosom. When the bosom disease has spread to the tissue outside your milk pipes, it can start to spread to another close by organs and tissue.

Invasive lobular carcinoma. Obtrusive lobular carcinoma (ILC) first creates in your bosom's lobules and is attacked close to tissue.

Other, more uncommon kinds of the bosom disease include:

Paget's illness of the areola. This kind of bosom disease starts in the conduits of the areola, however as it develops, it starts to influence the skin and areola of the areola.

Phyllodes cancer. This exceptionally uncommon sort of bosom disease fills in the connective tissue of the bosom. The majority of these growths are harmless, yet some are dangerous.

Angiosarcoma. This is a disease that develops in the veins or lymph vessels in the breast.

Breast cancer subtypes

Breast cancer growth is ordinarily additionally characterized in light of the surface proteins that are tracked down on the disease cells.

At the point when breast cancer growth tissue is eliminated from your body, it's tried for these proteins. The cancer growth cells are the subtypes in light of the presence or nonappearance of surface proteins. Knowing the subtype can assist your primary care physician in deciding the best course of therapy for your malignant growth.

How about we take a gander at the three most normal subtypes for bosom malignant growth?

Chemical receptor-positive
This subtype has estrogen and additionally progesterone receptors. An "emergency

room positive" growth has estrogen receptors, while a "PR positive" cancer has progesterone receptors. This subtype frequently needs chemicals compared to its receptors to develop.

It's assessed that around 70 percent of trusted Wellspring of bosom malignant growths are estrogen receptor-positive, while more than two-thirds of trusted Wellspring of those are additionally progesterone receptor positive.

Therapy hostile to estrogen or against progesterone chemical treatment can obstruct cancer development and kill the malignant growth cells. On the off chance that there are no receptors, it's known as a "chemical receptor negative" growth.

HER2 positive

This subtype has additional duplicates of the HER2 quality, so it delivers an over-the-top development chemical called HER2. This chemical permits the disease to develop all the more rapidly.

Therapy ordinarily includes prescriptions that can slow the development of this chemical and kill the malignant growth cells.

Around 20 to 25 percent of trusted wellsprings of bosom malignant growths are HER2 positive.

Triple-negative
Malignant growths that don't have an emergency room, PR, or HER2 receptors, are classified as "triple negative".

It's more considered normal in ladies who have a BRCA1 quality.

Less common types of breast cancer

More uncommon sorts of bosom malignant growth are frequently named by how they look under a magnifying lens. Here is a more intensive glance at a few more uncommon sports.

Provocative bosom malignant growth (IBC)

Provocative bosom malignant growth is a quickly developing, forceful sort of bosom disease that has various side effects to most different kinds of bosom malignant growth. Since it doesn't present as an irregularity, IBC is frequently confused with different circumstances.

Probably the most widely recognized side effects of IBC include:

an enlarged, warm, red bosom

bosom skin that is thickened or pitted

warmest that feels bigger or heavier than typical

torment or delicacy in the bosom or encompassing region

irritation close by the bosom

a transformed areola

The side effects of IBC are brought about by a blockage of the lymphatic framework inside the bosom. These side effects will more often than not grow rapidly, for the most part within 3 to a half years.

Paget infection of the bosom

Paget sickness is an uncommon malignant growth that structures in the milk channels and spreads to the skin of the areola and areola, the skin around the areola. This sort of bosom malignant growth is generally joined by DCIS or intrusive cancer inside the bosom.

The side effects of Paget infection are frequently confused at first with skin conditions, similar to skin inflammation or dermatitis. Be that as it may, the side effects will not answer skin medicines.

The run-of-the-mill side effects of Paget infection include:

redness, chipping, or crusting around the areola and areola
shivering or tingling sensation around the areola region
thickened skin on or close to the areola
a straightened areola
horrendous or yellowish release from the areola

Phyllodes growths of the bosom

A phyllodes growth is an exceptionally interesting kind of bosom disease that records for under 1 percent trusted Wellspring of all bosom cancers

In around 75 percent of trusted Source cases, phyllodes growths aren't carcinogenic, so they for the most part don't spread past the bosom. In any case, they can develop rapidly and some can be thought of as "fringe," which implies they have properties that could make them carcinogenic at a later stage.

Phyllodes grow a structure in the connective tissue of the bosom. The most widely recognized side effects include:

a smooth protuberance in or around the bosom

a protuberance that develops rapidly and extends the skin
bosom skin that looks red

Cylindrical carcinoma of the bosom

Cylindrical carcinoma is a subtype of obtrusive ductal carcinoma (IDC). This sort of bosom malignant growth gets its name because of the cylinder-formed structures, which should be visible under a magnifying instrument, that make up cancer. The cancers are typically little (around 1 centimeter or less) and will more often than not develop gradually. They are interesting.

Since these cancers are little, they are most frequently distinguished during a standard mammogram. They will more often than not be poor quality with great visualization.

Mucinous (colloid) carcinoma of the bosom

Mucinous carcinoma, otherwise called colloid carcinoma, is an interesting type of invasive ductal carcinoma (IDC). Around 2% of bosom malignant growths are "unadulterated" mucinous carcinoma, while up to 7 percent of bosom diseases have some part of mucinous carcinoma cells.

With this kind of malignant growth, cancer comprises unusual cells that seem to "float" in pools of bodily fluid when checked under a magnifying lens out
Ordinarily, a less forceful sort of malignant growth has a lower likelihood of spreading to the axillary (underarm) lymph hubs than a few different kinds of IDC.

Mucinous carcinoma will in general be more normal in post-menopausal ladies, with the typical age at determination being around 60 to 70 years old.

Medullary carcinoma of the bosom
Medullary carcinoma of the bosom is another interesting subtype of intrusive ductal carcinoma (IDC). It represents around under 5% of all bosom malignant growth cases.

The growth is ordinarily a delicate, meaty mass as opposed to a protuberance in the bosom tissue. The mass is most frequently created in the bosom and is most frequently tracked down in ladies with the BRCA1 transformation.

Albeit these disease cells frequently have a forceful appearance, they don't develop rapidly and for the most part, don't spread to the lymph hubs. This makes it more

straightforward to treat than a few different
sorts of breast cancer growth

.

Chapter3

STAGES OF BREAST CANCER

Malignant growths that are enormous or have attacked close by tissues or organs are at a higher stage than diseases that are little or still contained in the bosom. To organize bosom malignant growth, specialists need to be aware:

•on the off chance that the malignant growth is intrusive or painless.
•how enormous the growth is
•whether the lymph hubs are involved
•on the off chance that the malignant growth has spread to local tissue or disease
Bosom malignant growth has five fundamental stages: stages 0 to 4.

Stage 0 breast cancer growth

Stage 0 is DCIS. Malignant growth cells in DCIS stay restricted to the conduits in the bosom and have not spread into neighboring tissue.

Stage 1 bosom malignant growth

Stage 1A. The essential cancer is 2 centimeters (cm) wide or less. The lymph hubs are not impacted.
Stage 1B. Malignant growth is tracked down in neighboring lymph hubs. Either there is no growth in the bosom, or the cancer is more modest than 2 cm.

Stage 2 breast cancer growth

Stage 2A. The growth is more modest than 2 cm and has spread to 1 to 3 close by lymph hubs, or it's somewhere in the range of 2 and 5 cm and hasn't spread to any lymph hubs.

Stage 2B. The growth is somewhere in the range of 2 and 5 cm and has spread to 1 to 3 axillary (armpit) lymph hubs, or it's bigger than 5 cm and hasn't spread to any lymph hubs.

Stage 3 bosom malignant growth

Stage 3A.
The malignant growth has spread to 4 to 9 axillary lymph hubs or has amplified the interior mammary lymph hubs. The essential growth can be any size.

Growths are more noteworthy than 5 cm. The malignant growth has spread to 1 to 3 axillary lymph hubs or any breastbone hubs.

Stage 3B. A growth has attacked the chest wall or skin and could conceivably have attacked up to 9 lymph hubs.

Stage 3C. Malignant growth is tracked down in at least 10 axillary lymph hubs, lymph hubs close to the collarbone, or interior mammary hubs.

Stage 4 breast cancer growth (metastatic bosom disease)

Stage 4 bosom malignant growth can have a cancer of any size. Its malignant growth cells have spread to neighboring and far off lymph hubs as well as far off organs.

The testing of your primary care physician will decide the phase of your bosom malignant growth, which will influence your treatment.

Chapter 4

RISK FACTORS FOR BREAST CANCER

tracked down in ladies more than 55 years of age.

Drinking liquor. Liquor use jumble raises your gamble.

Having thick bosom tissue. Thick bosom tissue makes mammograms hard to peruse. It additionally expands your gamble of bosom malignant growth.

Orientation. As indicated by the ACSTrusted Source, white ladies are multiple times more bound to foster bosom malignant growth than white men, and Individuals of color are multiple times bound to foster bosom disease than Individuals of color.

Qualities. Individuals who have the BRCA1 and BRCA2 quality transformations are bound to foster bosom malignant growth more than individuals who don't. Other quality transformations may likewise influence your gamble.

Early feminine cycle. On the off chance that you had your most memorable period before you were 12 years of age, you have an expanded gamble of bosom malignant growth.

Conceiving an offspring at a more established age. Individuals who have their most memorable youngster following 35 years of age have an expanded gamble of bosom malignant growth.

Chemical treatment. Individuals who took or are taking postmenopausal estrogen and progesterone prescriptions to assist with diminishing their indications of menopause side effects have a higher gamble of bosom malignant growth.

Acquired risk. On the off chance that a nearby female relative has had bosom malignant growth, you have an expanded gamble of creating it. This incorporates your mom, grandma, sister, or little girl. On the off chance that you don't have a family background of bosom malignant growth, you can in any case foster bosom disease. A great many people who foster it have no family background of the infection.

Late menopause start. Individuals who start menopause after they're 55 years of age are bound to foster bosom malignant growth.

Never having been pregnant. Individuals who have never become pregnant or conveyed a pregnancy to full term are bound to foster bosom malignant growth.

Past bosom malignant growth. On the off chance that you have had bosom malignant growth in one bosom, you have an expanded gamble of creating bosom disease in your other bosom or an alternate region of the recently impacted bosom.

Chapter5

PREVENTION OF BREAST CANCER

While there are risk factors you have zero control over, following a solid way of life, getting customary screenings, and going to any preventive lengths your primary care physician suggests can assist with bringing down your gamble of creating bosom malignant growth.

Way of life factors

Way of life variables can influence your gamble of bosom malignant growth.

For example, individuals who have corpulence have a higher gamble of creating bosom malignant growth. Keeping a supplement-thick eating regimen and getting customary activity as frequently as conceivable could assist you with shedding pounds and lowering your gamble.

As indicated by the American Relationship for Malignant growth Exploration, liquor abuse additionally expands your gamble. This can have multiple beverages each day or hit the bottle hard.

On the off chance that you drink liquor, talk with your primary care physician about what sum they suggest for you.

Bosom malignant growth screening
Having customary mammograms may not forestall bosom malignant growth, however, it can assist with diminishing the opportunity that it will go undetected.

The American School of Doctors (ACP) gives the accompanying general suggestions to ladies at normal gamble of bosom malignant growth:

Ladies ages 40 to 49. A yearly mammogram isn't suggested, however, talk about your inclinations with your primary care physician.
Ladies ages 50 to 74. A mammogram every other year is suggested.
Ladies 75 years and more established. Mammograms are not generally suggested.
The ACP likewise advises against mammograms for ladies with a future of 10 years or less.

These are just rules.

Suggestions from the ACSTrusted Source contrast. As indicated by the ACS, ladies ought to:

have the choice of getting yearly screenings at 40 years of age

start yearly screenings at 45 years of age

move to screen every year at 55 years of age

Explicit suggestions for mammograms are different for everybody, so talk with your primary care physician to check whether you ought to get customary mammograms.

Preventive treatment

You might have an expanded gamble of bosom malignant growth because of inherited factors.

For example, on the off chance that your parent has a BRCA1 or BRCA2 quality transformation, you're at a higher gamble of having it too. This fundamentally raises your gamble of bosom malignant growth.

On the off chance that you're in danger of this transformation, talk with your primary care physician about your demonstrative and prophylactic treatment choices. You might need to be tried to see if you have the transformation.

Furthermore, assuming you discover that you in all actuality do have it, talk with your primary care physician about any precautionary advances you can take to decrease your gamble of creating bosom malignant growth. These means could incorporate a prophylactic mastectomy or careful evacuation of a bosom. You may likewise consider chemoprophylaxis, or taking a prescription, like Tamoxifen, to possibly diminish your bosom malignant growth risk.

Notwithstanding mammograms, bosom tests are one more method for looking for indications of bosom malignant growth.

Self-tests

Many individuals do a bosom self-assessment. It's ideal to do this test one time each month, simultaneously every month. The test can assist you with getting comfortable with how your bosoms generally look and feel so that you're mindful of any progressions that happen.

Remember, however, that the ACSTrusted Source believes these tests to be discretionary because ebb and flow research hasn't shown an unmistakable advantage of actual tests, whether performed at home or by a specialist.

Bosom test by your primary care physician
Similar rules for self-tests given above are consistent with bosom tests done by your primary care physician or other medical services proficient. They won't hurt you, and

your primary care physician might do a bosom test during your yearly visit.

On the off chance that you're having side effects that worry you, it's really smart to have your primary care physician do a bosom test. During the test, your primary care physician will check both of your bosoms for unusual spots or indications of bosom malignant growth.

Your primary care physician may likewise actually take a look at different pieces of your body to check whether the side effects you're having could be connected with another condition.

Chapter6

TREATMENT OF BREAST CANCER

Our bosom's malignant growth stage, how far it has attacked (on the off chance that it has), and how enormous cancer has developed all have a huge impact on figuring out what sort of therapy you'll require.

To begin, your primary care physician will decide your malignant growth's size, stage, and grade. Your disease's grade portrays that it is so liable to develop and spread. From that point forward, you can talk about your treatment choices.

The medical procedure is the most widely recognized therapy for bosom malignant growth. Many individuals have extra therapies, like chemotherapy, designated treatment, radiation, or chemical treatment.

Medical procedure

A few sorts of a medical procedures might be utilized to eliminate bosom malignant growth, including:

Lumpectomy. This methodology eliminates the growth and some encompassing tissue, leaving the remainder of the bosom in salvageable shape.

Mastectomy. In this methodology, a specialist eliminates a whole bosom. In a twofold mastectomy, they eliminate the two bosoms.

Sentinel hub biopsy. This medical procedure eliminates a couple of the lymph hubs that get seepage from the growth. These lymph hubs will be tried. On the off chance that they don't have malignant growth, you may not require an extra medical procedure to eliminate more lymph hubs.

Axillary lymph hub analysis. On the off chance that lymph hubs eliminated during a sentinel hub biopsy contain malignant growth cells, your primary care physician might eliminate extra lymph hubs.

Contralateral prophylactic mastectomy. Even though bosom malignant growth might be available in only one bosom, certain individuals choose to have a contralateral prophylactic mastectomy. This medical procedure eliminates your sound bosom to bring down your gamble of creating bosom malignant growth once more.

Radiation treatment

With radiation treatment, powerful light emissions are utilized to target and kill malignant growth cells. Most radiation therapies utilize outside pillar radiation. This procedure utilizes an enormous machine outwardly of the body.

Progress in malignant growth therapy has additionally empowered specialists to illuminate disease from inside the body. As indicated by Breastcancer.org, this kind of radiation therapy is called brachytherapy.

To direct brachytherapy, specialists place radioactive seeds, or pellets, inside the body close to the growth site. The seeds stay there for a brief timeframe and attempt to obliterate malignant growth cells.

Chemotherapy

Chemotherapy is a medication therapy used to obliterate malignant growth cells. Certain individuals might go through chemotherapy all alone, however, this kind of treatment is frequently utilized alongside different medicines, particularly medical procedures.

Certain individuals will have a medical procedure previously followed by different therapies, for example, chemo or radiation. This is called adjuvant treatment. Others might have chemotherapy first to contract the malignant growth, called neoadjuvant treatment, then, at that point, a medical procedure.

Now and again, specialists like to give chemotherapy before a medical procedure. The expectation is that the treatment will contract cancer, and afterward, the medical procedure won't be as intrusive.

Chemotherapy makes numerous undesirable side impacts, so talk about your interests with your primary care physician before beginning treatment.

Chemical treatment
On the off chance that your kind of bosom malignant growth is delicate to chemicals, your primary care physician might begin

you on chemical treatment. Estrogen and progesterone, two female chemicals, can invigorate the development of bosom malignant growth cancers.

Chemical treatment works by obstructing your body's development of these chemicals or by hindering the chemical receptors on the malignant growth cells. This activity can help slow and conceivably stop the development of your malignant growth.

Extra prescriptions
Certain therapies are intended to go after unambiguous inconsistencies or transformations inside malignant growth cells.

For instance, Herceptin (trastuzumab) can obstruct your body's development of the HER2 protein. HER2 assists bosom disease cells with developing, so taking a prescription to slow the creation of this protein might assist with easing back malignant growth development

.

Chapter7

BREAST CANCER TREATMENT BY STAGE

Stage 0 (DCIS)

On the off chance that precancerous or malignant growth cells are restricted to the milk channels, it's called a painless bosom disease or ductal carcinoma in situ (DCIS).

Stage 0 bosom malignant growth can become intrusive and spread past the channels. Early therapy can prevent you from creating intrusive bosom malignant growth. Early therapy can incorporate medical procedures like lumpectomy and mastectomy followed by radiation.

Stage 1

Stage 1A bosom malignant growth implies the essential cancer is 2 centimeters or less and the axillary lymph hubs aren't impacted. In stage 1B, malignant growth is found in lymph hubs and there's no cancer in the bosom of the cancer is more modest than 2 centimeters.

Both 1A and 1B are viewed as beginning phase intrusive bosom malignant growths. Medical procedures and at least one different treatment, similar to radiation or chemical treatment, might be suggested.

Stage 2

In stage 2A, the growth is more modest than 2 centimeters and has spread to somewhere in the range of one and three close-by lymph hubs. Or on the other hand, it's somewhere in the range of 2 and 5 centimeters and hasn't spread to lymph hubs.

Stage 2B means the cancer is somewhere in the range of 2 and 5 centimeters and has spread to somewhere in the range of one and three close-by lymph hubs. Or on the other hand, it's bigger than 5 centimeters and hasn't spread to any lymph hubs.

You'll most likely need a blend of a medical procedure, chemotherapy, and at least one of the accompanying: designated treatment, radiation, and chemical therapy.

Stage 3
Treatment for stage 3 ordinarily includes a blend of medicines including:

Foundational treatments. Foundational treatments incorporate chemotherapy, designated treatment for HER2-positive malignant growths, and chemical treatment for chemical receptor-positive diseases.
Medical procedure. If malignant growth improves with chemo, the subsequent stage is a medical procedure. Since IBC is so

forceful and influences an enormous region of the bosom and skin, bosom-moderating medical procedures like lumpectomies and incomplete mastectomies are impossible. All things being equal, medical procedure ordinarily includes the evacuation of the whole bosom through a changed revolutionary mastectomy. If malignant growth doesn't answer chemotherapy, medical procedure isn't possible and other chemotherapy medications or radiation treatment will be utilized.

Radiation treatment. Radiation therapy given after a medical procedure, called adjuvant radiation, can bring down the possibilities that malignant growth will return.

Stage 4

Individuals with stage 4 are fundamentally treated with foundational treatment, even though medical procedures and radiation might be choices in specific circumstances. Foundational treatment might include:

chemotherapy
hormonal treatment (for chemical receptor-positive malignant growths)
designated treatment (for HER2-positive malignant growths)
Provocative bosom malignant growth treatment
Provocative bosom malignant growth (IBC) is an unprecedented and forceful kind of bosom disease brought about by malignant growth cells obstructing lymph vessels in the skin.

All IBC cases are delegated essentially stage 3 bosom malignant growth. On the off chance that the malignant growth is metastatic (has spread to different pieces of the body), it's viewed as stage 4.

Therapies for IBC rely upon what stage the malignant growth is in.

HEALTHLINE Asset
Shared Bosom Malignant growth Stories and that's only the tip of the iceberg
Tap into local area discussions talking about bosom malignant growth analysis, supported by our strong BC people group. Bezzy BC: enabled by one another.

Immunotherapy as an arising treatment

Immunotherapy is a moderately new therapy choice, and keeping in mind that it hasn't been supported by the Food and Medication Organization (FDA) for bosom malignant growth yet, it's a promising region.

Immunotherapy works by raising the body's regular protection to ward off malignant growth. It has fewer incidental effects than chemotherapy and is less inclined to cause obstruction.

Pembrolizumab is an insusceptible designated spot inhibitor. A kind of immunotherapy has shown specific commitment to the therapy of metastatic bosom malignant growth.

It works by obstructing explicit antibodies that make it harder for the insusceptible framework to battle malignant growth. This permits the body to productively retaliate more. A recent report found that 37.5 percent of patients with triple-negative bosom malignant growth saw advantages from the treatment.

Since immunotherapy isn't FDA-supported at this point, treatment is for the most part accessible through clinical preliminaries as of now.

Corresponding and elective medicines

Certain individuals with bosom malignant growth may be keen on investigating corresponding or elective medicines like nutrients, spices, needle therapy, and back rub.

These therapies are utilized closely by conventional bosom malignant growth treatments to treat disease or free malignant growth side effects and awkward aftereffects from medicines like chemotherapy. You can investigate these therapies at any phase of bosom malignant growth.

Chapter8

FACTORS IMPACTING BREAST CANCER TREATMENT

While the breast cancer growth stage has a great deal to do with treatment choices, different variables can influence your treatment choices too.

Age

The visualization for breast cancer growth is generally more regrettable in individuals more youthful than 40 since the bosom disease will in general be more forceful in more youthful individuals.

Offsetting self-perception with saw risk decrease might assume a part in the choice between lumpectomy and mastectomy.

Notwithstanding medical procedures, chemotherapy, and radiation, quite a long while of hormonal treatment for chemical-positive bosom malignant growths is frequently suggested for youngsters. This can assist with forestalling a repeat or spread of bosom malignant growth.

For premenopausal individuals, ovarian concealment might be prescribed notwithstanding chemical treatment.

Pregnancy
Being pregnant additionally influences breast cancer growth treatment. Breast cancer growth medical procedure is generally alright for individuals who are pregnant, however, specialists might beat

chemotherapy until the second or third trimester down.

Chemical treatment and radiation treatment can hurt an unborn child and aren't suggested during pregnancy.

Cancer development
Therapy additionally relies heavily on how quickly the malignant growth develops and spreads.

On the off chance that you have a forceful type of bosom malignant growth, your primary care physician might suggest a more forceful methodology, like a medical procedure and a blend of different treatments.

Hereditary qualities and family ancestry

Therapy for bosom malignant growth might rely part of the way upon having a direct relation with a background marked by breast cancer or testing positive for a quality that expands the gamble of creating breast cancer growth.

Patients with these variables might pick a preventive careful choice, like a reciprocal mastectomy.

Clinical preliminaries

Clinical preliminaries are concentrated in which patients volunteer to attempt new medications, blends of medications, and strategies for treatment under the cautious management of specialists and scientists. Clinical preliminaries are a significant stage in finding new bosom malignant growth treatment strategies.

Arising therapies for bosom malignant growth being concentrated on in clinical preliminaries include:

PARP inhibitors that block proteins used to fix DNA harm that happens during cell division are being utilized and tried for TNBC.
Drugs that block androgen receptorsTrusted Source or forestall androgen creation are being utilized and tried for TNBC.

www.ingramcontent.com/pod-product-compliance
Lightning Source LLC
Chambersburg PA
CBHW051704250726
48653CB00007B/2837